AF797412

Dr. Del's RAPID FATLOSS

Detox-Cleanse Program

A 21-Day Whole Food Based Plan for Jumpstarting Your Body's Fat-Burning System.

Features:

- *The 21-Day Detox-Cleanse Meal Plan*
- *Dr. Del's Top Ten SuperFoods*
- *Weekly Menu's & Shopping Lists*

Del Millers, PhD

Author of:

- *Dr. Del's Rapid Fatloss Manual*
- *Dr. Del's Rapid Fatloss Meal Plan*
- *Dr. Del's Rapid Fatloss Cookbook*
- *Dr. Del's Rapid Fatloss Detox-Cleanse Program*
- *Simply DELicious: 10-Minute Meals Cookbook*
- *Del's 10-Minute Workout*
- *Dancing with God*

Dr. Del's Rapid Fatloss Detox-Cleanse Program
A 21-Day Whole Food Based Plan for Jumpstarting Your Body's Fat-Burning System

Del Millers, PhD

Published by

Spiritwind Publications
10736 Jefferson Blvd., # 693
Culver City, CA 90230 U.S.A.
888-800-9463

All rights reserved. No part of this book may be reproduced or transmitted in any form or by any means, electronic or mechanical, including photocopying, recording or by any information storage and retrieval system without written permission from the author, except for the inclusion of brief quotations in a review.

Copyright © 2012
by Del Millers, PhD

Publisher's Cataloging-in-Publication Data

Millers, Del.
Dr. Del's rapid fatloss detox-cleanse program : a 21-day whole food based plan for jumpstarting your body's fat-burning system / Del Millers.
p. cm.
ISBN: 978-0-96667045-5
1. Weight loss. 2. Detoxification (Health). 3. Diet therapy. I. Title.
RM222.2 .M5246 2012
613.2`5—dc22
2012904104

Design by Linda Björk
Photographs Michael Burr

Printed in the United States of America

Dedicated to all the members
and future members of the
Living Lean club.

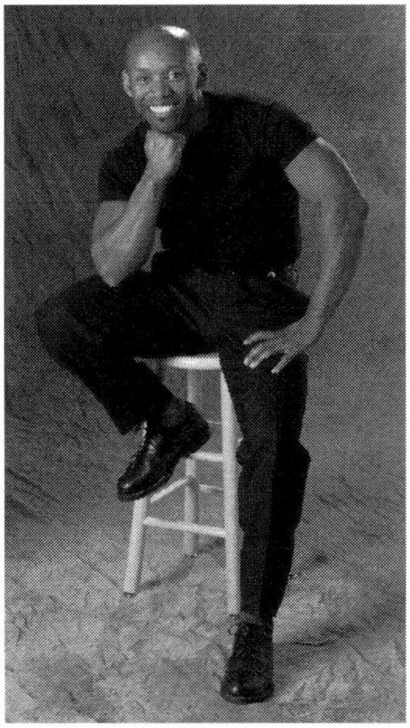

"True silence is the rest of the mind;
it is to the spirit what sleep is to the body,
nourishment and refreshment."
~ *William Penn*

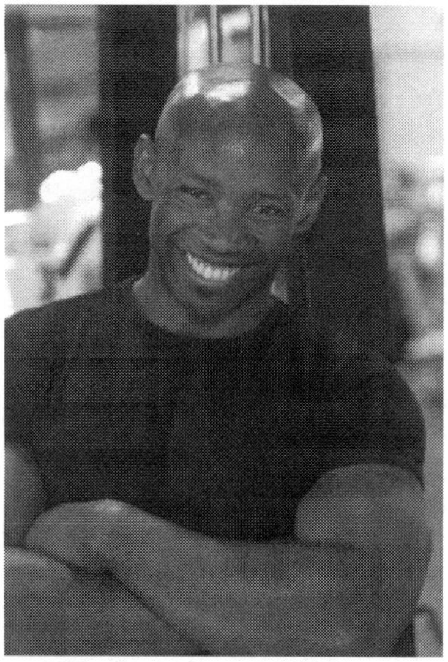

Dr. Del's Personal Mission Statement:

To Inspire, Support and Encourage
Personal Growth & Transformation
through Health Conscious Living.

Table Of Contents

The 21-Day Detox-Cleanse Program

Obesity, high blood pressure, high cholesterol, etc. are all bi-products of the body not being healthy. Therefore, the very first phase of my 3-phase nutrition program with most of my clients is to focus on improving their health.

I said most of my clients because not all are willing or ready to totally give up the junk that they eat, which brings up a very important point.

If you can't function without your daily sugar and caffeine fix, then that should tell you something about yourself; you have lost the ability to make conscious choice.

Without the ability to consciously choose what and when you eat, you no longer have any control over your body or your health.

The focus of this 21-day detox-cleanse program is to restore your ability to make conscious choice, and to get the body's various systems functioning optimally.

If you are addicted to sugar, caffeine and other addictive substances, then the only way to break the cycle of addiction is to first stop the behavior.

Why is this important?

You will never transform your body and your health if you have no control over what you eat. I'm not talking here about deprivation. I'm talking about conscious eating.

You don't have to deprive yourself of the pleasure of eating your treats to get great results. To be successful, however, you have to be able to consciously decide when to eat treats and when not to.

If you don't have the discipline to decide that you're not going to eat something for the next few weeks because it's not part of your plan right now, then you will always be a slave to your cravings.

The purpose of this 21-Day Detox-Cleanse Program is to help you break the cycle of unconscious eating and reprogram your taste buds. This is important because if you simply try to cut back on the junk that you've been eating, you will fail. You have to first give up everything for a while and reclaim your power of choice.

Now, before you scream, "No, not again!" don't fret. You'll have my cookbook with dozens of healthy meals that are quick and easy to make, and most importantly, they taste fantastic.

Plus, detoxifying your body isn't what it sounds like—you'll likely be eating more food, in far richer variety during these 21 days than you have in the past.

You'll enjoy rich grains and delectable fruits. Vitamin-packed all natural smoothies and some of the best soups you've ever tasted. And best of all, you'll be making them yourself—as easy as these meals are, they're perfect for the creative chef buried deep inside you.

If nothing else, during this 21-Day Detox period, you'll learn how to play with your food and make it taste great.

So what exactly will happen to your body during this detox period?

The point of detoxifying your body is to give it only what it needs to improve and maximize bodily functions and rid itself of the toxins that have built up throughout the past due to poor eating and lifestyle habits.

The only items you'll sacrifice during this period are what I call *The Five White Poisons.*

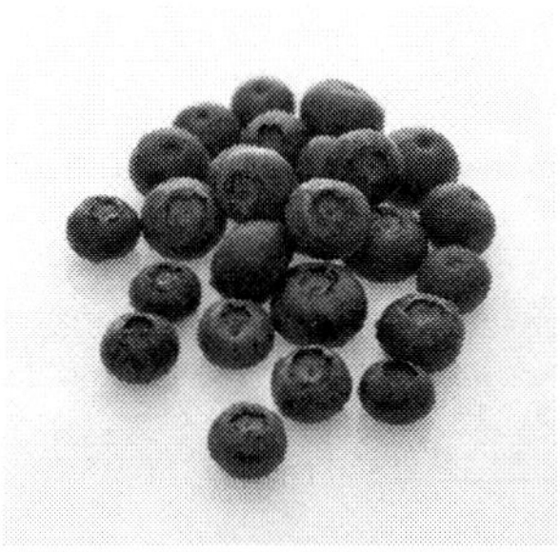

The Five White Poisons:

❶ White Flour:
Unbleached "enriched" flour has been stripped of all its nutritional value and adds nothing to your body's health.

❷ Table Salt:
All 70 naturally occurring minerals have been processed out (sea salt is a better option).

❸ Milk/Dairy Products:
Most people are lactose intolerant, though they may not even know it. Besides, dairy often is the cause of excessive mucus production in the body.

❹ Refined Sugar & Artificial Sweeteners:
We can easily understand why sugar, as a simple carbohydrates, is not beneficial to your health and body transformation goals. The worst thing you could do is substitute artificial sweeteners.

I never recommend anything artificial or man-made. Besides, there are conflicting research data on whether artificial sweeteners pose a health risk. But do you really want to put your health in the hands of people who only care about how much money they can make?

❺ Alcohol and Caffeine:
Too much alcohol and caffeine interfere with many of your body's natural functions and cause your liver and kidneys to work overtime to rid you of their toxin byproducts. Alcohol & caffeine may even caused the body to become deficient in certain important fat burning nutrients.

Instead of the above, we will feed the body only natural whole foods (grains, legumes, fruits and vegetables, healthy essential fats) and lots of water.

At the end of this first phase of the program, you will feel a significant increase in energy, vibrancy, increased bowel movement and, of course, an average weight/fat loss of 5-15 pounds.

Supplementation

You will use a fruit and vegetable capsule JuicePlus® 3x/day—before breakfast, before lunch and before dinner with a glass of water--and take Essential Fatty Acid fish oil supplements 2x per day to give the body an abundance of raw material to neutralize and flush out built up toxins.

In short, this process is critical to enabling your body to once again become the muscle building, fat burning, energy-generating machine that it was meant to be. I also encourage the use of milk thistle extracts and probiotics to aid in digestion.

This dietary approach is especially helpful for those who regularly experience fatigue, gastrointestinal problems and food and environmental sensitivities.

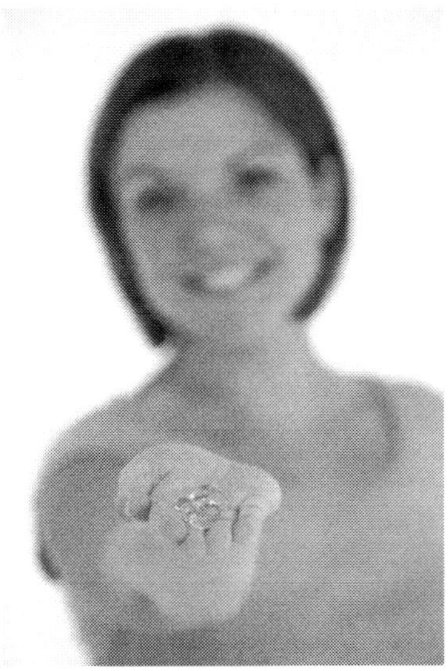

Raw vs. Cooked Foods

Did you know that whether your food is raw or cooked can make a difference in how much of it is absorbed by the body?

Let's take tomatoes for example. Tomatoes are rich in a compound called lycopene, a form of antioxidant believed to protect against prostate cancer. However, while fresh tomatoes have a total antioxidant potential of about 80, cooked tomatoes have about six times as much lycopene.

Scientists believe that this happens because when cooked the lycopene is transformed to trans-lycopene, which is much more readily absorbed by the body, hence, more bioavailable.

Bioavailability refers to the quantity or fraction of a particular ingested nutrient that is absorbed into the bloodstream. There are many factors that affect bio-availability such as age, health status, food interaction, metabolism, among others. Therefore, nutrients from food are never fully absorbed into the blood-stream.

Like tomatoes, carrots, kale and other hard vegetables are more bioavailable when cooked. By slightly cooking these vegetables you break down the hard cellulose fiber, thus, releasing more of the nutrients (antioxidants).

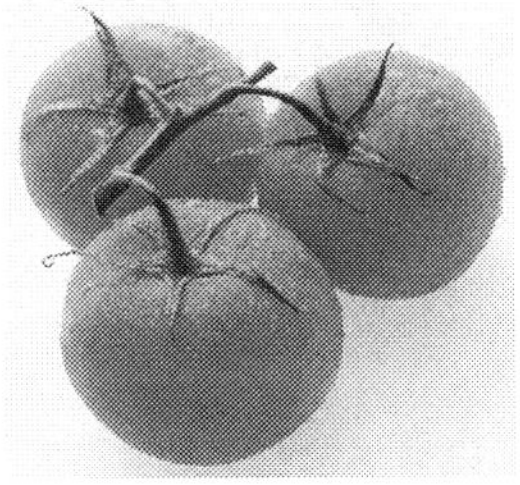

Fat vs. Water-Soluble Nutrients

Did you also know that eating certain nutrients with a little fat could make the difference in how well they're absorbed by the body (how bioavailable they are)?

Let's take lutein for example, found in kale, spinach, broccoli and peas. Lutein is a "fat-soluble" nutrient that helps protect against macular degeneration (a leading cause of blindness in older people).

However, in order for the body to properly absorb lutein, and other fat-soluble nutrients, it has to first get them out of their cellular structure (light cooking helps), then they have to be attached to lipophillic (fat-loving) carriers in the stomach to be absorbed into the bloodstream.

Conclusion. Cooking your dark green leafy vegetables with a little oil (such as stir-frying or steaming them then adding a drop of oil) will help your body to absorb the fat-soluble nutrients better.

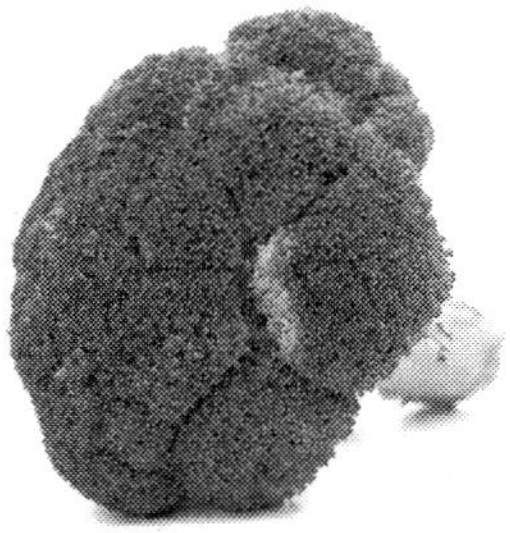

Some Basic Nutrient (Food) Combinations

Food combination and how the body absorbs nutrients is a very complicated science. For this reason I recommend eating an array of "whole foods" everyday of different colors. The different colors represent different classes of nutrients.

As mentioned before, adding a whole food supplement like Juiceplus fruit and vegetable capsules, which contains ALL the nutrients from 17 raw, vine-ripened, mostly all organic fruits and vegetables, minus the sugar, salt and water to your daily regime is beneficial.

I use this product because it's the only one of it's kind that I know of that's been tested to be bioavailable. And now you understand the importance of bio-availability.

As you can see, without the right balance of nutrients, you may be eating the right foods, however, your body may not be absorbing enough of the nutrients because other co-nutrients are missing.

Food	Nutrient	Benefit	Why it works
Spinach & Orange Juice	Iron	Prevents anemia, energy loss & infections	Vitamin C helps the body to absorb more iron from vegetables
Cooked Tomatoes	Lycopene	Prevents cell damage & prostate cancer	Cooking increases lycopene content of tomatoes six times
Cooked dense fibrous vegetables (i.e. carrots)	Beta carotene & others	Antioxidants	Cooking breaks down the hard cellulose fiber, releasing more nutrients
Leafy vegetables & oil	Lutein & others	Prevent various diseases	Oil aids in absorption of fat-soluble nutrients

Keep in mind that there are pros and cons to food combination. For example, cooking tomatoes to increase the lycopene content will degrade the vitamin C content. For this reason, I highly recommend eating a variety of some lightly cooked vegetables and eating others raw.

The bottom line:

On my 21-Day Detox-Cleanse Program you'll come to appreciate the importance of eating a variety of fruits and vegetables daily; some cooked and some raw.

This is important because it's the little things that make the biggest difference to your health. What I mean is you're not always aware of the thousands of "micro-nutrients" and other plant chemicals present in plant foods that are vital to your health.

Yet, if you don't eat enough of them your body may become deficient in other nutrients because it may not have the ability to absorb them from your foods. The obvious conclusion is to always make sure that you eat a rainbow of colors each day.

The different colors of plant foods represent different classes of nutrients, but they all work together synergistically to help you build your best body from the inside out.

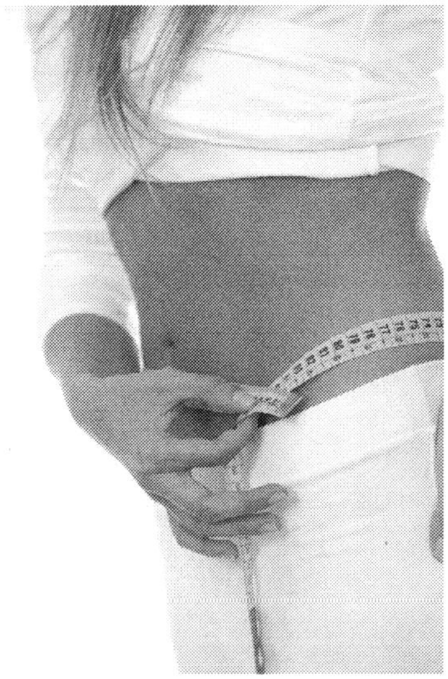

Death Begins in the Colon

Are you feeling sluggish, bloated, or stressed? Are your skin and eyes lacking the glow and sparkle, which come with healthy living? Maybe it's time to consider a detox/cleanse!

Let me begin by asking you a simple question, "How many bowel movements do you have per day?"

Yes, by bowel movements I mean a number two. Now if you answered, "I have as many bowel movements as meals," then pat yourself on the back, you're on the right track. Any less than that and you're constipated!

Would you believe that most Americans can't go to the bathroom without laxatives? Well, believe it because it's true. In fact, I've worked with clients who barely had one bowel movement per week...talk about being "full of shit!"

Why is it important to maintain a healthy colon?

Let me ask you this? When was the last time you changed the oil in your car? Would you go an entire year without changing the oil in your car? How about five or ten? I think not.

The liver and colon is the "sewage system" of the body. And within the colon walls there live a host of bacteria (some good, some bad, and some down-right ugly), parasites and other debris.

If plaque can form on your teeth based on what you eat, don't you think the same plaque, or worse, can also form within the colon, thereby creating blockage, and in some cases, re-absorption of waste matter into the blood-stream?

I hope your answer is yes, because the truth is, "death begins in the colon." This is why the rate of colon cancer has dramatically increased by over 40% in the past few decades.

Remember, the human Gastrointestinal (GI) track consists of the esophagus, stomach, small intestine, and colon/large intestine. Undigested foods cannot be absorbed into the walls of the small intestine to enter the bloodstream, therefore they are sent down the track to the large intestine (colon) as waste to be re-absorbed after being acted upon by special enzymes and bacteria or eliminated as feces.

If waste cannot be re-absorbed and it is not eliminated, just imagine what would happen in your colon if it just sits there month after month, year after year. If you've ever used a public toilet, I'm sure you've entered a stall where someone forgot to flush...it wasn't a pretty site was it. And I'm sure it didn't smell much better. You get the point.

If you're not yet convinced why a colon/intestinal cleanse is important, I think you'd better check your pulse.

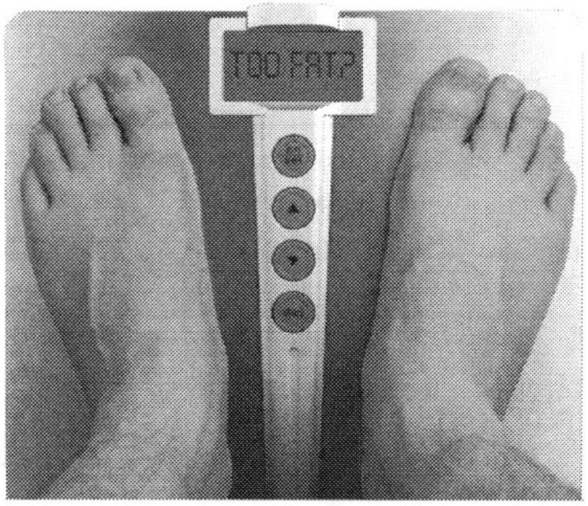

How Do I Detox the Liver & Colon?

The idea behind detoxing is simple. You cut foods containing harmful chemicals from the diet, while flushing out the impurities already in the body by drinking a lot of filtered or mineral water.

However, keep in mind that detoxing is really only sensible if it's part of a longer-term plan. You are deluded if you think you can make up for 11 months' slacking with one month's abstinence.

Our bodies, specifically our livers, work overtime to rid themselves of the toxins - or at least unnecessary substances - we put through them daily, including pesticides and growth hormones in our food, alcohol, tobacco, caffeine and hard-to-digest substances like dairy products.

Eating an abundance of whole foods, some raw and some cooked, and limiting the amount of chemicals we put into the body allows the liver and colon to "cleanse" themselves of the impurities we ingest on a daily basis.

By cooking all our meals from the freshest, most nutritious ingredients, we revive our bodies and help eliminate the cravings for processed foods.

Apart from cutting out the consumption of alcohol and caffeine, you must also stay clear of refined foods, such as white sugar, white rice, and highly processed foods such as instant meals and snacks, which are full of stabilizers, preservatives, colorings and other artificial food additives, beef, pork, butter and all saturated fats, hydrogenated oils, cigarettes and recreational drugs.

It's also crucial to cut out meat, the residues of which can clog up the intestines for months, dairy products, and wheat products such as bread, pasta and couscous.

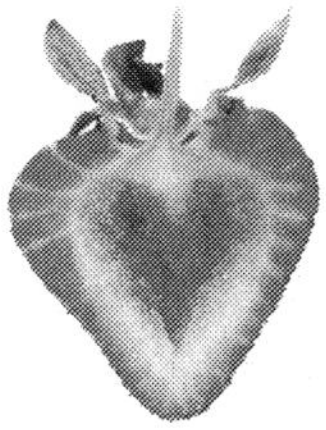

Will Herbs Help?

If you do decide to detox, your liver will be your body's main cleansing organ, filtering around two liters of blood per minute and removing 99% of bacteria and toxins from the blood before releasing it back into the body.

In addition to flushing the body through with at least a gallon of filtered or mineral water a day, you must also replace alcoholic drinks, tea and coffee with fresh-squeezed fruit juice, fruit tea and herbal teas.

Herbs will not only help to clean and scrub, but also draw out old fecal matter and toxins, stop bleeding, disinfect, kill and expel parasites, kill Candida albicans overgrowth (which is a major contributor towards Irritable Bowel Syndrome and Crohns disease), regulate and balance intestinal flora, remove toxic metals (such as lead, mercury, radioactive metals) and strengthen the muscles of the colon to promote normal bowel movements (and therefore heal spastic colon).

Some herbs or spices to aid digestion, calm alimentary canal conditions such as infections and inflammations and help flush the system through.

Peppermint, spearmint and ginger teas - available in bag form from supermarkets and health food shops – may aid digestion and act as mild antiseptics.

Artichoke leaf (available in capsule form) may also aid digestion.

Better digestion will mean that toxins aren't being absorbed into the body.

To boost the liver, try *milk thistle* (available from health food shops or herbalists). *Oat bran and ground oats* are also valuable detox tools.

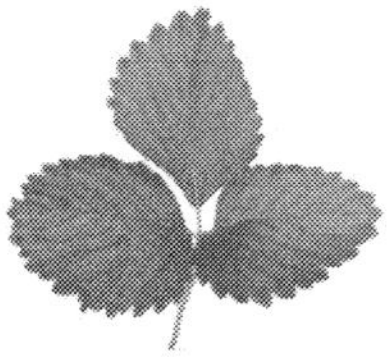

Probiotics

Probiotics (good bacteria) can also make a huge difference as they are an essential part of digestion. Many of us don't have all the good bacteria we should because of antibiotics and because our environment and farming practices are so far removed from nature.

Many people believe that often problems that don't appear to be related to the colon will in many cases improve with colon cleansing. After all, when you step on a cat's tail, it's the other end that screams.

Toxins cause pain and disease. And a dirty bowel is full of toxins.

Besides, a lot of extra waste material inside will over work your organs.

Yes, I do recommend a detox/cleanse to my clients. That's why it's the first phase of my three -phase nutrition program. The complete program is outlined in ***Dr. Del's Rapid FatLoss Manual.***

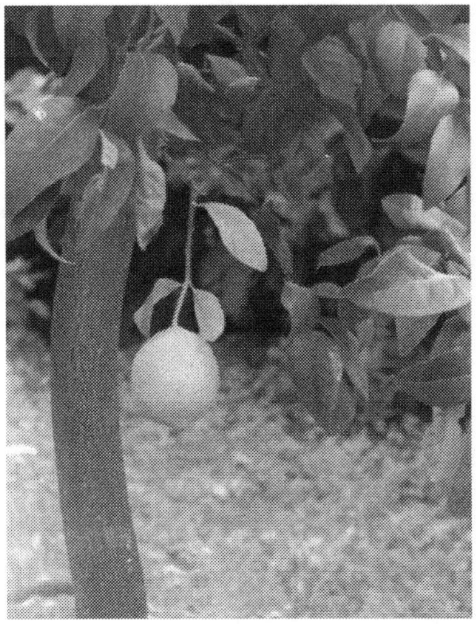

Dr. Del's Top Ten Superfoods

Below is my list of the top ten foods that should be on your shopping list every week and why. However, this is not to say that other plant foods are of lesser importance; that is not the case. Every plant food has nutritional value and the important thing to remember is that all nutrients work in synergy.

In fact, individually, they can do nothing. That is why I have always advocated eating a rainbow of colors because each color represents a different set of nutrients that must be combined with other nutrients to be absorbed into the bloodstream.

▼ Dark Green Leafy Vegetables
(Kale, Spinach, broccoli, collard greens, etc.)

Dark green leafy vegetables contain thousands of plant substances (lutein, flavonoids, folic acid, vitamins C and E, and fiber) that have been shown to prevent various disease conditions in the body.

▼ Berries **(blackberries, blueberries, raspberries, strawberries, etc.).**

Berries are among the fruits highest in antioxidant content and are excellent sources of several phytochemicals that seem to help block cancer development.

Anthocyanins, Ellagic acid and Pterostilbene are just a few of the powerful phytochemicals found in all berries. These compounds have been shown to inhibit the growth of lung, colon and leukemia cancer cells without affecting the growth of healthy cells. They also affect metabolic processes to decrease development of both cancer and heart disease.

When selecting berries, note that the darker they are, the more anti-oxidants they have.

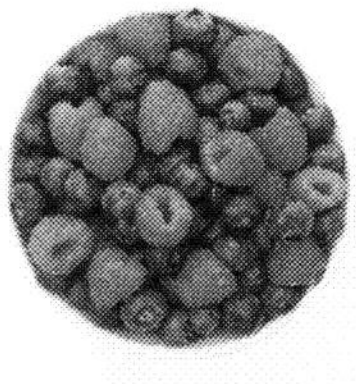

▼ Oats

Oats are very high fiber cereal grains. Oats, oat bran, and oatmeal contain a specific type of fiber known as beta-glucan. Since 1963, several studies have proven the beneficial effects of this special fiber on cholesterol levels.

Studies show that in individuals with high cholesterol (above 220 mg/dl), consuming just 3 grams of soluble oat fiber per day (an amount found in one bowl of oatmeal) typically lowers total cholesterol by 8-23%.

This is highly significant because each 1% drop in serum cholesterol translates to a 2% decrease in the risk of developing heart disease. High cholesterol levels correlate with the build up of plaques in blood vessel walls.

If these plaques become damaged or simply grow too large, they can rupture, blocking a blood vessel and causing a heart attack, stroke, or blood clots elsewhere in the body. Lowering high cholesterol levels can therefore significantly reduce the risk of cardiovascular disease and stroke.

Oats are available in several forms. Oat groats are the whole seed with only the outer hull removed. Rolled oats are the familiar breakfast form. Steel cut oats are oat seeds that have been chopped into pieces.

Quick Oats are rolled steel cut oats, and instant oats are pre-cooked, dried and flattened steel cut oats.

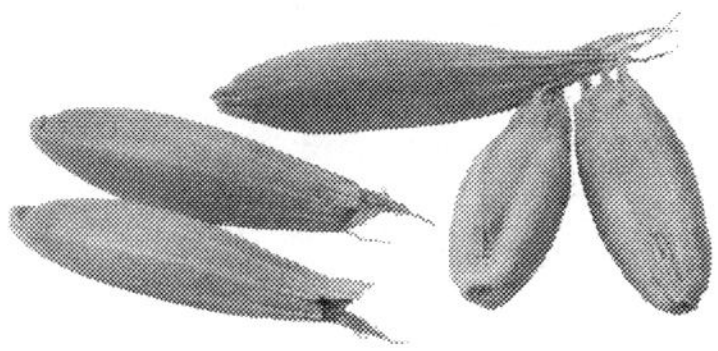

▼ Beans

Beans are a good source of several nutrients, including iron, protein, B vitamins, folic acid and oil or starch. Beans with colored shells contain antioxidants. They are a rich source of fiber, which helps to reduce levels of LDL cholesterol in blood.

Fiber is also known as 'roughage' and is important because it absorbs water, adds bulk and ensures that wastes pass out of the body efficiently. If this does not happen several problems can occur including constipation and diverticular disease.

Soybeans are the stars of the bean world. They are the only beans to contain all eight amino acids necessary to make a 'complete' protein. They also contain phytoestrogens, which are thought to slow bone loss; reduce the chances of prostate cancer and heart disease.

▼ Wild omega 3-rich fish

Omega-3 fats found mostly in wild fatty fish lowers your risk of heart disease, help arthritis, and may possibly help with memory loss and Alzheimer's disease, according to various studies. These heart-healthy fats may even help to reduce depression as well.

Omega-3's are most prevalent in fatty, cold-water fish. Look for wild (not farmed) salmon, herring, sardines, and mackerel. Aim for two-to-three servings a week. Other forms of omega-3's are available in flax seeds, and walnuts.

These superfoods have the added benefit of being high in monounsaturated fats, which can lower cholesterol.

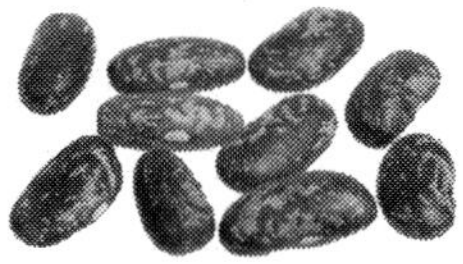

▼ Tea (white, green & black)

Until recently, tea research has focused on green tea. Green tea is loaded with the compound epigallocatechin gallate (EGCg), a powerful antioxidant. However, new research has also discovered that both black and white teas contain high levels of flavonoids, which helped reduce the production of LDL - the "bad" cholesterol that can lead to stroke and heart attacks.

Furthermore, men who drank over four cups of black tea per day had a significantly lower risk of stroke than men who drank only two to three cups per day. All the above mentioned teas are also rich sources of catechins, another group of powerful antioxidants.

▼ Soy

To eat soy or not to eat soy — that seems to be the question on many people's minds these days. What are we to make of all this conflicting information about the benefits and dangers of soy? Let's settle this issue once and for all.

For 5,000 years soy has been considered one of the five sacred plants (in China) — the others being rice, wheat, barley and millet. Soy is a non-animal protein that contains all eight of the essential amino acids, making it the only complete plant protein. Whole soy foods also are a good source of fiber, B vitamins, calcium, and omega-3 fatty acids.

In 1999, the FDA allowed soy food manufacturers to advertise the health claim that 25 grams of soy protein a day could reduce bad cholesterol (LDL) levels. This claim did not extend to isolated isoflavones. Shortly thereafter, a backlash of research was soon published purporting that soy was a dangerous allergen, created thyroid problems and caused cancer.

The negative studies on soy isoflavones have used isolated compounds containing isoflavone amounts that far exceed what a person would normally eat and have tested these substances on mice, which metabolize soy very differently from humans (just as dogs cannot tolerate chocolate), and arrived at what I feel are dubious if not erroneous conclusions about the dangers of soy.

However, a well-balanced August 2005 report from the Agency for Health-care Research and Quality reviewed hundreds of studies with support from the National Institute of Health. In the 68 studies examining the impact of soy on cholesterol levels, they found that it did indeed reduce LDL and triglyceride levels. They found insufficient data among 200 human studies to suggest that soy had an effect — negative or positive — on bone health, cancer, kidney disease, endocrine function, reproductive health, neurocognitive function, or glucose metabolism.

Organic edamame, tofu and soymilk are the best form of soy to eat.

▼ Nuts & Seeds

Nuts are one of the best plant sources of protein. They are rich in fiber, phytonutrients and antioxidants such as Vitamin E and selenium. Nuts are also high in plant sterols and fat - but mostly monounsaturated and polyunsaturated fats (omega 3 - the good fats), which have all been shown to lower LDL cholesterol.

In addition to nuts, seeds such as flax seeds, pumpkin seeds and sunflower seeds may offer the same heart health benefits. Research conducted at the Harvard School of Public Health, the Iowa Women's Healthy Study and the Physician's Health Study have all shown that people who ate nuts 2-4 times per week had reduced risks of sudden cardiac death and 40% lower risks of heart disease.

▼ Tomatoes

Although they are thought of as a vegetable, tomatoes are botanically classified as fruits. They are also one of our best sources of vitamin C. Tomatoes also contain an abundance of lycopene, which helps support immune function and prostate health. Cooked tomatoes found in pasta sauce, salsa and tomato paste enhance the absorption of lycopene into your system.

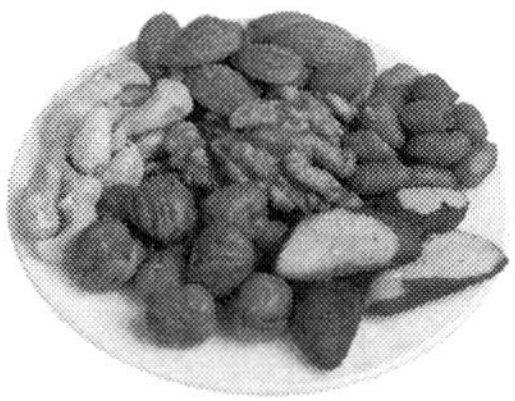

▼ Garlic

Garlic is one of the oldest known medicinal plants, and it's been credited with fighting heart disease, lowering blood pressure and helping to fight off colds. Studies suggest that individuals regularly consuming garlic show a lower incidence of stomach cancer, have longer blood clotting times and show lower blood lipid levels (which indirectly translates into reduced risk of stroke and cardiovascular disease).

The anti-bacterial properties of garlic also help the body to fight off infections.

▼ The bottom-line

I have chosen this group of ten foods because they have been shown to have the highest concentration of disease-fighting nutrients. However, please keep in mind that the wide range of phytochemicals found in fruits, vegetables, whole grains and legumes act together in ways far greater than would be expected from looking at them individually. That's why, as fabulously healthy as each of these foods are, you should always strive to add new ones to your diet regularly.

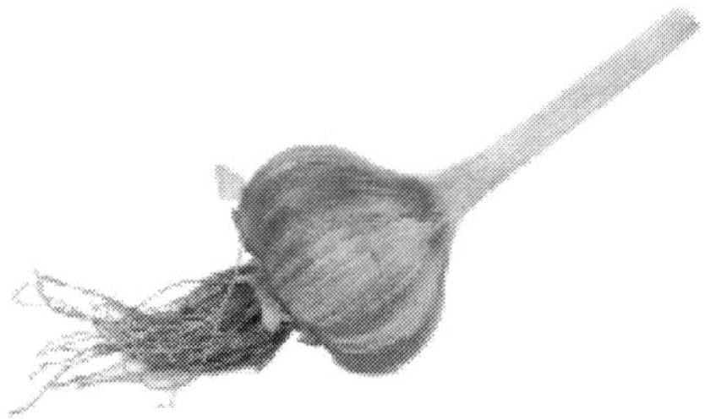

The 21-Day Detox-Cleanse Meal Plan

General Nutrition Guidelines

Eat in Abundance

ORGANIC FRUIT — fresh apricots, berries, kiwi, lemons, papaya, peaches, mango, grapes and melons. These fruits are naturally high in antioxidants and the amino acid glutathione. Glutathione conjugates with toxins in plasma before being converted into mercapturic acid, which can then be excreted via the kidneys.

In addition, all berries act as potent blood purifiers. Strawberries also play a role in helping to cleanse the lungs; they contain elagic acid, which reduces the effect of the carcinogen PAH, which is found in tobacco smoke.

Melons (particularly honeydew and cantaloupe) are packed with minerals, antioxidants and phytonutrients, all of which support the liver and balance the metabolism. Watermelon acts as a diuretic and has a strongly alkalizing effect (non-acidic) on the body.

Avoid grapefruit and grapefruit juice, which contain a compound called naringinin that can significantly inhibit liver enzymes involved in detoxification.

ORGANIC VEGETABLES — artichokes, beets, all leafy green vegetables, carrots, capsicums, cauliflower, cucumber, pumpkin, sweet potato, watercress, bean sprouts and broccoli. All these vegetables are alkalizing and high in antioxidants, essential minerals and dietary fiber.

In addition, artichokes contain plant compounds known as caffeoylquinic acids, which increase the flow of bile and help to digest fats. Beets contain betaine, which promotes the regeneration of liver cells and the flow of bile. Betaine also has a beneficial effect on fat metabolism. Broccoli and other brassicas (cabbage, kale, etc.) support the liver's detoxification enzymes.

Foods to Eat in Moderation

The following foods make detoxing easier by providing extra energy and important amino acids.

GRAINS — organic brown rice, corn, millet and quinoa. No more than two portions a day.

OILY FISH — wild salmon, mackerel, sardines, tuna.

NUTS AND SEEDS — one handful a day of raw, organic, unsalted nuts and seeds. Choose from almonds, Brazils, hazelnuts, pecans, pumpkin seeds, sunflower seeds, sesame seeds and flax seeds. (Avoid if allergic.)

OILS — use a little organic extra virgin olive oil for cooking in place of butter or margarine. Use cold-pressed seed oils for dressings.

Drink Up

Water is vital because it helps to flush waste through your system. Drink at least 10-16 large glasses of filtered, bottled or spring water daily. Sip it slowly through the day rather than drinking with meals (which can dilute digestive juices). You should, however, drink a glass of water along with your fruit and vegetable capsules before each meal.

If you enjoy hot beverages try herbal teas and dandelion "coffee." Both are alternatives to caffeine and can actively help detoxing. For example, dandelion is a natural diuretic and an overall tonic for the liver and digestive tract.

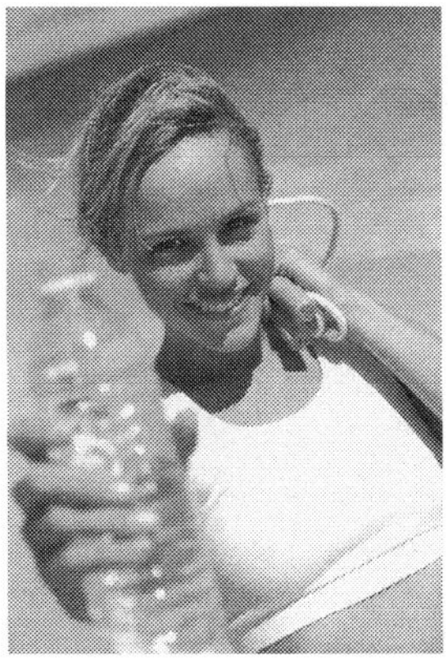

Foods to Avoid During Your Detox

Avoid the following:

- All wheat products (bread, pasta, cake, cookies, muffins, cereals, etc.)
- Meat, and dairy products (milk, cheese, butter, cream)
- Salt and any foods containing it
- Sugar (cakes, candy, cookies, etc.) and artificial sweeteners (aspartame, saccharin, etc.)
- All processed and fast food
- Foods containing additives and preservatives
- Hydrogenated fats
- Alcohol and caffeine (this includes tea--green/black teas are okay-- and sodas)
- Gluten--Avoid all foods that contain wheat, spelt, kamut. This include bread, pasta, cereals, crackers and any product containing flour.
- Red meat, chicken, turkey and any meat products like sausages, burgers, and pate
- Milk, cheese, cream
- Butter and margarine
- Any food that contains wheat including bread, croissants, cereals, cakes, biscuits, pies, pastry, quiche, battered or bread crumbed foods, etc
- Crisps and savory snacks including salted nuts
- Chocolate, sweets, jam and sugar
- Processed foods, ready meals, ready-made sauces and takeaways
- Alcohol
- Coffee and tea (green tea is okay).
- Sauces, pickles, shop bought salad dressing, mayonnaise
- Salt
- Fizzy drinks and squashes, including diet versions

Best Sources of Protein

Cold water fish:
- *Wild Pacific or Atlantic Salmon*
- *Halibut*
- *Cod*
- *Sole*
- *Trout*
- *Haddock*
- *Pollock*
- *Mackerel*

Tofu
Legumes (beans, peas, lentils)
Egg whites
Salmon/tuna canned
Edamame
Organic Almond/Soy Milk (Unsweetened)
Hummus

Best Sources of Complex Carbohydrates

Sweet potato
Brown/wild rice
Millet
Buckwheat
Gluten-free products
- *bread*
- *pasta*

Quinoa
Amaranth
Oats
Vegetables (all vegetables--fresh, frozen or freshly squeezed)
Fruits (all fresh whole fruits in season)

Best Sources of Fats & Oil (cold pressed)

Canola
Olive (extra virgin)
Sesame
Seeds: sesame, flax, pumpkin
Nuts: almonds, walnuts pecans
Almond butter
Tahini (ground sesame seeds)

Meal Replacement:

JuicePlus Complete

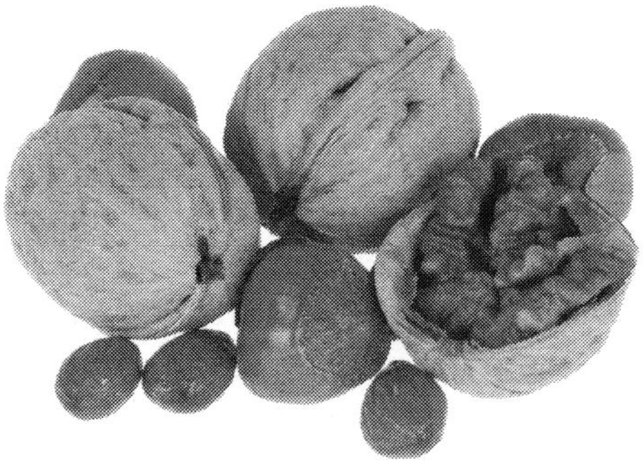

Detox-Cleanse Meal Plan Summary

Food Group	Allowed	Avoid
Protein	Cold water fish: - Wild Pacific or Atlantic Salmon - Halibut - Cod - Sole - Trout - Haddock - Pollock - Mackerel Tofu Legumes (beans, peas, lentils) Egg whites Salmon/tuna canned Edamame Organic Almond/SoyMilk (Unsweetened) Hummus	Red Meats Cold cuts Poultry Sausages
Complex Carbohydrates	Sweet potato Brown/wild rice Millet Buckwheat Gluten-free products - bread - pasta Quinoa Amaranth Oats Vegetables (all vegetables-fresh, frozen or freshly squeezed) Fruits (all fresh whole fruits in season)	All gluten containing products...pasta, bread, all non-gluten-free baked goods, ketchup, salad dressings, etc.
Dairy	Live-cultured plain yogurt	Milk, cheese, all other dairy products
Fats, Nuts & Seeds	Canola Olive (extra virgin) Sesame Seeds: sesame, flax, pumpkin Nuts: almonds, walnuts, pecans Almond butter Tahini (ground sesame seeds)	Margarine, other vegetable oils, salad dressings
Beverages	Green/black tea, freshly squeezed vegetable juices	Coffee, alcohol, soda, all sweetened beverages

Basic Salad Dressing

3 tbsp lemon juice
4 tbsp sesame or extra virgin olive oil
1 clove crushed garlic
1 tsp dijon mustard
A dash of oregano, basil, thyme or sea salt

❶ Mix all ingredients together and refrigerate. Shake well before serving.

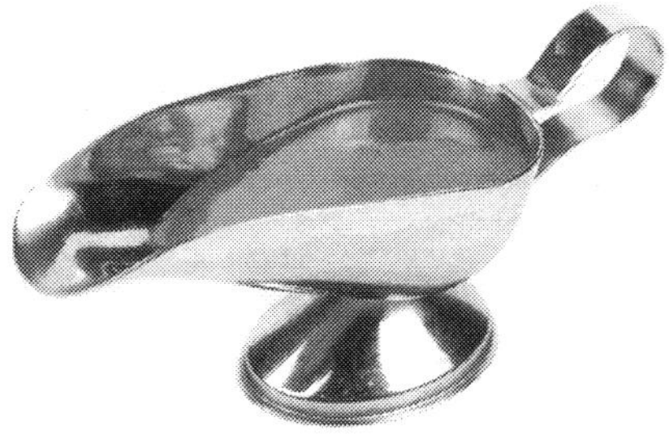

21-Day Detox-Cleanse 3-Week Menu

Week 1

Meal	Day 1	Day 2	Day 3	Day 4	Day 5	Day 6	Day 7
Breakfast	1/2 cup Oatmeal 2 egg whites 1 egg 1 tsp almond butter Juiceplus Fruit Fish Oil	Protein smoothie: 1/4 cup oatmeal 1 cup fruit 1 tsp almond butter 1 cup soymilk (unsweetened) JuicePlus Fruit Fish oil	Egg white scramble 1 egg, 2 whites medium tomato 1/2 small avocado 1 piece fruit JuicePlus Fruit Fish oil	1/2 cup oatmeal 2 egg whites 1 egg 1/2 cup berries 1 tsp peanut butter Juiceplus Fruit Fish oil	Blueberry-mango-banana smoothie (RFCookbook) Juiceplus Fruit Fish oil	Scrambled Egg Whites with Tomato Basil & Avocado (Simply Delicious) Juiceplus Fruit Fish oil	Choose any detox plan meal
Lunch	Tuna & Sweet Corn Salad (Simply Delicious) Juiceplus Vineyard	1 cup veggie soup Tuna salad: Spinach 1/4 cup beans 2 egg whites 3-oz tuna Juiceplus Vineyard	Raw vegetable & bean salad Juiceplus Vineyard	Curried brown rice salad Juiceplus Vineyard	Tuna w/ tomato & avocado salad (Simply Delicious) Juiceplus Vineyard	Ginger Orange Tofu & Spinach Brown rice (Simply Delicious) Juiceplus Vineyard	
Afternoon	1 cup chopped fruit 1/2 cup plain yogurt 6 almonds	chopped veggies 2 tbsp hummus	1 cup plain yogurt 1 cup fruit 1 tsp oats 6 almonds	1 piece fruit 1 tsp almond butter	3 egg whites 1 tsp almond butter 1 fruit	Berrilicious Smoothie (RFCookbook)	
Dinner	Orange Zest Salmon (RF-Cookbook) 1 cup veggies 1/4 small avocado Juiceplus Veggie Fish oil	Sweet & sour stir fry w/rice Juiceplus veggie Fish oil	Lime-ginger Pan Seared Sole (RFCookbook) 1 cup veggies Juiceplus veggie Fish oil	Lemon-Ginger Trout (Simply Delicious) Juiceplus veggie Fish oil	Honey Mustard Snapper (Simply Delicious) Juiceplus veggie Fish oil	Spicy Tofu & Asparagus with Garlic Ginger Sauce (Simply Delicious) Juiceplus veggie Fish oil	

Week 2:

Meal	Day 1	Day 2	Day 3	Day 4	Day 5	Day 6	Day 7
Breakfast	Toasted Oatmeal with Apples, Almonds & Banana (RFCookbook) Juiceplus Fruit Fish oil	Strawberrilicious Smoothie (RFCookbook) JuicePlus Fruit Fish oil	Spinach-tomato egg white scramble (RFCookbook) 1 piece fruit JuicePlus Fruit Fish oil	Breakfast Bowl (RFCookbook) Juiceplus Fruit Fish oil	Yogurt Parfait (RFCookbook) Juiceplus Fruit Fish oil	Scrambled Egg Whites with Tomato, Basil & Avocado (RFCookbook) Juiceplus Fruit Fish oil	Choose any detox plan meal
Lunch	Arugula Salad w/Figs & Walnuts (RFCookbook) Juiceplus Vineyard	Escarole & White Bean Soup (RFCookbook) Juiceplus Vineyard	Seared Ahi Tuna Salad w/Wasabi Vinaigrette (RFCookbook) Juiceplus Vineyard	Tofu-Carrot-Ginger Soup (RFCookbook) Juiceplus Vineyard	Three-Bean Salad (RFCookbook) Juiceplus Vineyard	Smoked Salmon with Edamame (RFCookbook) Juiceplus Vineyard	
Afternoon	1 cup chopped fruit 1/2-cup plain yogurt 6 almonds	Peanutty hummus & sliced apple (RFCookbook)	1 cup plain yogurt 1 cup fruit 1 tsp oats 6 almonds	1 piece fruit 1 tsp almond butter	3 egg whites 1 tsp almond butter 1 fruit	Berrilicious Smoothie (RFCookbook)	
Dinner	Cod w/chili, garlic, ginger sauce (RFCookbook) 1 cup veggies 1/4 small avocado Juiceplus Veggie Fish oil	Sweet & sour stir fry w/rice Juiceplus veggie Fish oil	4 oz fish 1 cup veggies Juiceplus veggie Fish oil	Lemon Ginger Trout (Simply Delicious) Juiceplus veggie Fish oil	Honey Mustard Snapper (Simply DELicious) Juiceplus veggie Fish oil	Spicy Tofu & Asparagus with Garlic Ginger Sauce (Simply Delicious) Juiceplus veggie Fish oil	

Week 3:

Meal	Day 1	Day 2	Day 3	Day 4	Day 5	Day 6	Day 7
Breakfast	Toasted Oatmeal with Apples, Almonds & Banana (RFCook-book) Juiceplus Fruit Fish oil	Hard Boiled Egg Whites & Fruit (RFCook-book) JuicePlus Fruit Fish oil	Spinach-tomato egg white scramble (RFCook-book) 1 piece fruit JuicePlus Fruit Fish oil	Breakfast Bowl (RFCook-book) Juiceplus Fruit Fish oil	Yogurt Parfait (RFCook-book) Juiceplus Fruit Fish oil	Scrambled Egg Whites with To-mato, Basil & Avocado (RFCook-book) Juiceplus Fruit Fish oil	Choose any detox plan meal
Lunch	Tuna with Apple, Tomato & Avocado Salad (RFCook-book) Juiceplus Vineyard	Pan-Seared Tofu Wrap w/Orange Chili Sauce (RFCook-book) Juiceplus Vineyard	Seared Ahi Tuna Salad w/Wasabi Vinaigrette (RFCook-book) Juiceplus Vineyard	Tofu-Carrot-Ginger Soup (RFCook-book) Juiceplus-Vineyard	Three-Bean Salad (RFCook-book) Juiceplus Vineyard	Smoked Salmon with Edamame (RFCook-book) Juiceplus Vineyard	
Afternoon	1 cup chopped fruit 1/2-cup plain yogurt 6 almonds	Peanutty hummus & sliced apple (RFCook-book)	1 cup plain yogurt 1 cup fruit 1 tsp oats 6 almonds	1 piece fruit 1 tsp almond butter	3 egg whites 1 tsp almond butter 1 fruit	Berrilicious Smoothie (RFCook-book)	
Dinner	Cod w/chili, garlic, ginger sauce (RFCook-book) 1 cup veggies 1/4 small avocado Juiceplus Veggie Fish oil	Sweet & sour stir fry w/rice Juiceplus veggie Fish oil	Brazilian Black Bean Stew (RFCook-book) 1 cup veggies Juiceplus veggie Fish oil	Lemon-Ginger Trout (Simply Deli-cious) Juiceplus veggie Fish oil	Honey Mustard Snapper (Simply DELicious) Juiceplus veggie Fish oil	Spicy Tofu & Asparagus with Garlic Ginger Sauce (Simply Deli-cious) Juiceplus veggie Fish oil	

Weekly Shopping List

Shopping List	Precooked	Pantry necessities
Salmon fillet Halibut Frozen shrimp Eggs Greek plain nonfat yogurt Soft silken tofu Firm tofu Mild salsa Rice paper wrappers (Asian market) Tahini	Brown rice Oatmeal	Black-eyed peas Canned tuna Canned salmon Canned black beans Canned kidney beans Canned white beans Canned pinto beans Canned lentils Old fashioned oats Soymilk (unsweetened) Raisins Protein Powder (JuicePlus Complete) Ground flax meal Peanut/almond butter Sliced almonds Canned diced tomatoes Tomato paste Natural muesli (no sugar) Sesame seeds
Fruits & Vegetables: Apples Oranges Bananas Strawberries Spinach Tomatoes Avocado Red bell pepper Garlic Onions Green onions Large head of lettuce Mushrooms Cilantro Ginger Broccoli Potato Peach Ripe mango Sweet potato Shiitake mushroom		**Freezer:** Strawberries Blueberries Raspberries Shrimp Organic mixed vegetables Sweet corn Mango **Refrigerator:** Miso paste Pickled ginger

Detox-Cleanse Recipes:

The recipes for the meals listed on the Detox-Cleanse Meal Plan are either below or outlined in one of my cookbooks:

1. *Dr. Del's Rapid Fatloss Cookbook*
2. *Simply DELicious*

Detox Plan Breakfasts

▶ Oatmeal
Hot Oatmeal with Cinnamon & Nutmeg
(Recipe in the Rapid FatLoss Cookbook)

▶ Fruit salad with yogurt and oats
Fresh fruit salad with natural plain yogurt (1/2 cup), 1 tsp crushed nuts and a sprinkling (1 Tbsp) of oats.

▶ Fresh fruit & Tofu smoothie
1/2 banana, 1/2 cup berries, 1/4 cup raw oatmeal, 4 oz soft tofu 1 cup or water, 4 ice cubes, 1 tsp. flaxseed oil or flaxmeal. Blend.

▶ Homemade Muesli and yogurt
Homemade muesli made from 1/4 cup oats, 1 tsp. seeds, 1 tbsp. raw nuts and 1/4 cup dried fruit served with natural plain yogurt. Add cinnamon and nutmeg to taste.

▶ Scramble egg whites with Tomato & avocado
(Recipe in the Rapid FatLoss Cookbook)

▶ Scrambled tofu with tomato & avocado
(Recipe in the Rapid FatLoss Cookbook)

Detox Plan Lunches

▶ Vegetable soup

Large bowl of vegetable or lentil soup (either homemade or supermarket 'fresh') .

▶ Tuna and sweet corn salad

Tuna (canned in water) mixed with sweet corn and natural yogurt over mixed baby greens or spinach salad.

▶ Raw vegetable & Bean salad

3 hard boiled egg whites, 1 cup raw broccoli, 1 cup baby spinach, 1/2 cup white/pinto beans, 1 tbsp extra virgin olive or canola oil, 1 tbsp balsamic vinegar, 1/2 tsp. Dijon mustard, pepper, 1 tsp. natural unsalted raw nuts. Toss in a bowl.

▶ Eggless "Egg" Salad

8 oz. firm tofu mashed with a fork, 1 medium carrot (shredded), 2 chopped scallions, 1 tsp. Dijon mustard, 1 tsp. Mrs . Dash, pepper. Toss over salad greens.

▶ Three bean salad

1 tbsp. Red wine vinegar, 1 tbsp. Olive oil, 2 cloves garlic (minced), 1/2 medium red onion (chopped), 1/2 cup red kidney beans, 1/2 cup black beans, 1/4 cup white beans. Toss in a bowl.

▶ Curried brown rice salad

1 cup cooked brown rice, 1/2 cup broccoli, 1/4 cup chopped celery, 1/4 cup chopped red pepper, 1/2 red onion (chopped), 1/2 cup plain yogurt, 1 tbsp. Balsamic vinegar, 1 tsp. sesame oil, 1/2 tsp. curry powder, 1/2 tsp. Dijon mustard, Mrs. Dash & pepper to taste. Toss in a bowl.

▶ Tuna with Tomato & avocado salad

(Recipe in the Rapid FatLoss Cookbook)

▶ Ginger Orange Tofu & Spinach

(Recipe in the Rapid FatLoss Cookbook)

Detox Plan Dinners

▶ Chinese vegetable & Tofu Stir Fry
Stir fry a selection of vegetables such as bok choi, spring onions, mushrooms, bamboo shoots and bean sprouts with 8 oz firm tofu in a little olive oil with garlic and ginger. Serve with 1 cup brown rice.

▶ Lemon-Ginger Trout
(Recipe in the Rapid FatLoss Cookbook)

▶ Sweet and sour stir fry with rice
Gently fry a selection of chopped vegetables such as onions, peppers, baby sweet corn and mushrooms. Add 1/4 cup canned pineapple (in fruit juice), 1/2 cup canned tomatoes, tomato purée, 1 tbsp. white wine vinegar and honey. Bring to a boil and simmer until the sauce has thickened. Serve with brown rice.

▶ Zesty Orange sole fillets
(Recipe in the Rapid FatLoss Cookbook)

▶ Herb Salmon Fillet with Brown Rice and Steamed Kale
(Recipe in the Rapid FatLoss Cookbook)

▶ Black Beans with Ginger & Tofu
(Recipe in the Rapid FatLoss Cookbook)

▶ Curried swordfish with tropical fruit salsa
(Recipe in the Rapid FatLoss Cookbook)

Detox Plan Anytime Meals

- Fresh fruit or fresh fruit salad
- Natural plain yogurt mixed 1 tbsp. raw nuts and chopped fruit.
- Handful of unsalted nuts or seeds and a piece of fruit.
- Fruit smoothie (Rapid Fatloss Cookbook)
- 3 hard-boiled egg whites and 1 tbsp. almond butter

"If you don't like something change it;
if you can't change it,
change the way you think about it."
~ Mary Engelbreit

About the Author

Del Millers, Ph.D.
Author, Speaker, Life Coach

DEL THE AUTHOR

Other Books by Del Millers:

DR. DEL'S RAPID FATLOSS MANUAL:
A Scientific Approach to Building Your Leanest Body Ever

DR. DEL'S RAPID FATLOSS MEAL PLAN:
A Science Based Eating Strategy
for Building Your Leanest Body Ever.

DR. DEL'S RAPID FATLOSS COOKBOOK:
Quick & Easy "10-Minute Meals"
for Building Your Leanest Body Ever.

SIMPLY DELICIOUS:
Quick & Easy 10-Minute "Fit" Recipes
and Nutrition Guide.

DEL'S 10-MINUTE TOTAL BODY WORKOUT:
When all you've got is 10 minutes to spare!

DANCING WITH GOD:
How you can Make Exercise
a Playful Adventure of Body and Soul!

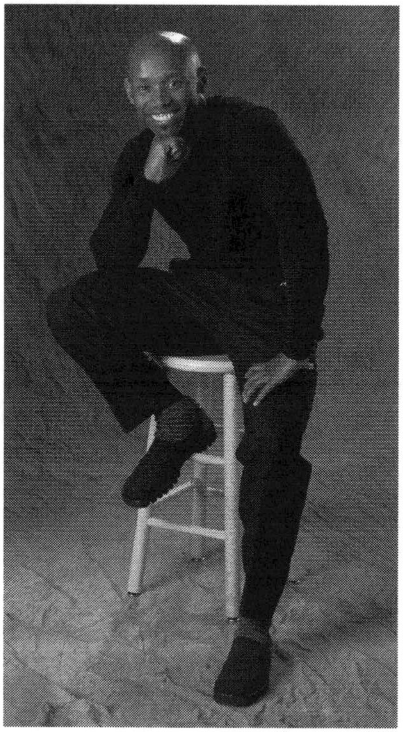

DEL THE SPEAKER

Speaking Engagements And Seminars:

Speaking the Spirit of the Body's Wisdom

When Del Millers speaks, people listen. He knows an awful lot about the physical body, and he looks like it. He also knows an awful lot about the mind and emotions, and he demonstrates it. And that he has a very intimate and personal relationship with his own spiritual nature puts him in a very unique position to be able to support, motivate, and encourage people to reach new levels with their personal dreams and ambitions. As one client puts it, "I have had many personal fitness trainers and many dance and tennis teachers. Del is the first one to really help me reach my goals. He's tough and demanding and kind at the same time. He knows what he's doing; he's an expert."

Del has been extremely successful as a motivational speaker and coach because he addresses all aspects of the human being. He is intelligent, well spoken, and engaging, whether he's exploring the many aspects of health and nutrition or describing how exercise is really like dancing with God. He fascinates audiences and individuals alike because he practices what he preaches. He is a happy man with a firm grasp on his reality—and he assists others to reach the same amazing place. He is, in a word, inspiring.

Del holds a Masters Degree in Spiritual Psychology, a degree he earned by demonstrating self-mastery, and a Ph.D. in Nutritional Sciences. He is also an accomplished writer, poet, and performer as well as a master instructor of Kung Fu and Tai Chi Chuan, a Personal Fitness Coach and a sought after corporate consultant. Del is truly a pioneer, combining the fields of Fitness and Transformation.

Del Millers is a powerhouse, standing on a solid foundation of education and experience. When he speaks, people want what he's got. The good news is, he knows how to deliver.

PRIVATE CONSULTATION

Dr. Del is available for phone or email fitness, nutrition and life coaching.

Del's Contact Information:

For consultations or to book Del for a seminar or speaking engagement, please contact:

DEL MILLERS

Del Millers International
10736 Jefferson Blvd. #693
Culver City, CA 90230
USA

http://www.delmillers.com
del@delmillers.com
1-888-800-9463

Subscribe to Dr. Del's FREE Email Newsletter:
www.drdelmillers.com

Subscribe to Dr. Del's Blog:
www.drdelblog.com

Dr. Del's Online Fitness & Nutrition Coaching Program:
Get a FREE Fitness Analysis and One-Month Membership
www.personalfitness.com

Join the conversation online:

FACEBOOK **Facebook.com/drdelmillers**
Like Dr Del for daily updates and postings

TWITTER **@drdelmillers**
Stay connected

YouTube **Youtube.com/drdelmillers**
Visit Dr. Del's video channel

DEL MILLERS INTERNATIONAL

Inspiration, Support & Encouragement,
For Your Personal Growth and Transformation!
http://www.delmillers.com

Made in United States
Troutdale, OR
07/25/2026

51590718R00027